Quick-Fire

General Surgery Review Questions & Topics

Bradley J. Phillips, MD

The Ranch
Author: *bjpmd2@aol.com*

from tragedy... Hope!

Table of Contents

        Section I

        Section II

        Section III

        Section IV

        Section V

        Section VI: Bonus 25 Questions

II.   **Review Topics**

        Acid-Base Disorders

        Hemodynamics

        Oxygen Calculations

        The Chest: pneumothorax, hemothorax, pleural effusions, & empyema

<u>Review Questions</u>

Section I: 50 Questions & Answers

Questions:

1. What is the most common complication of antrectomy ?

2. What are the three major components to MEN-I?

3. What is the most common cause of chronic cholestasis in children ?

4. What is the operation of choice in Achalasia ?

5. How do you diagnose a Gastrinoma ?

6. What is the most common site of obstruction from colon cancer ?

7. What is Boerhave's Syndrome ?

8. What is the most common neuroendocrine tumor found in MEN-I ?

9. What is the most common type of pituitary tumor found in MEN-I ?

10. How do you treat Toxic Megacolon ?

11. Which antibiotic has the highest incidence of producing *C. difficile* colitis ?

12. How do you treat a cecal volvulus ?

13. What chromosome is responsible for MEN-I ?

14. What is the usual cause of death in MEN-I patients ?

15. What is Ogilvie's Syndrome ?

16. What is a Cushing's Ulcer ?

17. What is MEN-II a?

18. What is MEN-IIb ?

19. What is the preoperative management of a patient with known pheochromocytoma ?

20. What is 'pancreas divisum' ?

21. How do you treat an annular pancreas ?

22. What is the 'normal' anatomy of the Left Recurrent Laryngeal Nerve ?

23. What is the 'normal' anatomy of the Right Recurrent Laryngeal Nerve ?

24. What are the most common causes of large bowel obstruction ?

25. How do you manage Crohn's disease of the appendix ?

26. What is a Type II Gastric Ulcer ?

27. What is the function of the External branch of the Superior Laryngeal Nerve ?

28. What is the function of the Internal branch of the Superior Laryngeal Nerve ?

29. How do you manage bile reflux gastritis ?

30. What is Plummer-Vinson Syndrome ?

31. How do you treat Gaucher's Disease ?

32. What is Hereditary Spherocytosis ?

33. How do you treat Hereditary Spherocytosis ?

34. Where does the Inferior Thyroid Artery originate?

35. What chromosome is BRCA-1 located on ?

36. What chromosome is BRCA-2 located on ?

37. What is a 'common' cause of massive hemoptysis in children ?

38. What is Ancanthosis nigracans ?

39. What is Horner's Syndrome ?

40. What is the "Blakemore Tube" and how is it used?

41. What factors are in Cryoprecipitate ?

42. What is the deficiency in Hemophilia A ?

43. What is the deficiency in Hemophilia B ?

44. What is the toxic dose of Lidocaine… with and without epinephrine ?

45. What is the classic sign of lidocaine toxicity ?

46. How do you calculate the Gradient in Portal Hypertension ?

47. How do you treat a Unilateral-locked facet ?

48. When do you give steroids for neuro-trauma ?

49. What are the three immune products of the spleen ?

50. What are Salter-Harris Classes and which ones may impede growth ?

Answers:

1. Bile reflux gastritis

2. "Werner's Syndrome":

   Parathyroid Hyperplasia
   Pancreatic Neuroendocrine Tumor
   Pancreatic Tumor

3. Congenital Biliary Atresia

4. Heller myotomy with or without Nissan fundiplication *(controversial)*

5. a. Serum Gastrin level > 500 ucg

   b. Basal acid output to maximal acid outout ratio > 0.6

   c. Calcium-stimulating test, 4 mg/ kg IV over 5 minutes: this will double the baseline gastrin level in the presence of a gastrinoma *(secretin stimulation is no longer performed)*

6. Sigmoid colon

7. Boerhave's is a post-emetic perforation of the esophagus which usually presents as fever and right-sided chest pain; early detection is the key to survival.

8. Gastrinoma

9. Prolactinoma

10. Treatment of toxic megacolon is dependent on the underlying state of the patient. Fluid resuscitation and intravenous broad-spectrum antibiotics are mandatory. If the patient is stable, you may consider urgent colonoscopic decompression (being careful not insufflate excessive air). If the pt is deteriorating or presents acutely unstable and actively septic, total abdominal colectomy may be necessary (in this situation, I would tend to perform a relatively quick operation utilizing an end-ileostomy rather than a primary anastamosis).

11. Clindamycin

12. Right hemicolectomy with ileocolic anastamosis; cecopexy is not preferred by most surgeons

13. Chromosome # 11

14. Neoplasia is the primary cause of death *(not the biochemical effects of the tumor)*

15. Colonic pseudo-obstruction which presents as massive abdominal distension

16. Stress ulcer associated with closed head injury

17. "Sipple's Syndrome":

    Parathyroid hyperplasia
    Pheochromocytoma
    Medullary Thyroid Cancer

18. Pheochromocytoma
    Medullary Thyroid Cancer
    Neuromas (as well as a marphinoid habitus)

19. To optimize medical management:
    a. 2 weeks preoperative - Alpha-blockade with Phenoxybenzamine

    b. 1 week preoperative - Beta-blockade with Inderal

    c. and, if necessary in the operating room – IV Phentolamine

20. Nonfusion of the Major (Wirsung) and Minor (Santorini) pancreatic ducts; the minor duct becomes the primary route of drainage

21. Duodenal bypass

22. Wraps around the aortic arch

23. Wraps around the right subclavian artery; the Right recurrent nerve has a more variable course compared to the Left

24. Large Bowel Obstruction: Carcinoma (2/3 of all)
    Volvulus
    Diverticular disease
    Hernias
    Intussusceptions
    Fecal impaction

25. Appendectomy if the cecum is not actively involved, otherwise may need to proceed with segmental resection. Remember, most fistulas do not arise from the appendiceal base but rather from the terminal ileum.

26. Type II is a gastric ulcer associated with a duodenal ulcer

27. Innervates the cricothyroid muscle to affect pitch

28. Sensory to the larynx

29. Surgical treatment of bile reflux:

    Convert B-I or B-II to a Roux-en-Y gastrojejunostomy with a 40 cm. jejunal distance

    Must ensure that there is a complete vagotomy and all of the antrum was previously resected

30. Esophageal webs, microcytic anemia, and smooth fingernails – which as a syndrome is associated with a higher risk of esophageal cancer*

31. partial splenectomy

32. autosomal dominant deficiency of spectrin leading to an inability of the red cell to deform appropriately which leads to splenomegaly and anemia

33. total splenectomy

34. the thyrocervical trunk

35. Chromosome # 17

36. Chromosome # 11

37. Tuberculosis *(treat by embolization)*

38. Bilateral axillary hyperpigmentation associated with underlying gastric ca or lung ca

39. Miosis, ptosis, anhydrosis

40. The Blakemore Tube: indicated in persistent UGI bleeding secondary to varices

    a.   Intubate the pt (you must secure the airway)
    b.   Place tube into the stomach
    c.   Inflate the gastric balloon with 50 cc's and confirm gastric position with KUB
    d.   After confirmation, inflate another 200 cc's
    e.   Place tube to 5lb's traction
    f.   If bleeding still persists, inflate Esophageal balloon to 40 mmHg

* remember, you must deflate the esophageal component every 12 hours to minimize wall ischemia and subsequent necrosis

41. Factor VIII, VonWillebrand's factor, and Fibrinogen

42. Factor VIII

43. Factor IX

44. The toxic dose of Lidocaine is between 5–7 mg/kg; with epinephrine the total dose injected is a bit higher secondary to local vasoconstriction.

A 1 % solution will contain 10 mg/cc.

a. With Epinephrine: 6 - 7 mg/kg in a 70 kg male
  =   420 – 470 mg total dose
  =   42 – 47 cc's injected

b. Without Epinephrine: 5 mg/kg in a 70 kg male
  =   350 mg total dose
  =   35 cc's injected

45. Seizures

46. Gradient = Wedged Hepatic P – Free Hepatic P
    (4-6 mmHg) *(5 – 10 mmHg)*   *(0 – 5 mmHg)*

    a.   Remember, only half of all cirrhotics will develop varices, and of these, only half will bleed (still adds up to major morbidity & mortality)

    b.   The role of surgery in Portal Hypertension, is only AFTER all medical and endoscopic measures have been taken

47. You must reduce a unilateral-locked facet with 5 lbs. of traction per vertebrae

48. Steroids in c-spine trauma remain controversial. They are never given for closed head injury! With c-spine injury (usually blunt), they are best if administered within 6 hrs of the traumatic mechanism. Solumedrol 30 mg/kg IV bolus followed by 5.4 mg/kg IV gtt for 23 hrs.

49. Tuftsin, properidin, and IgM

50. Salter-Harris I - V:

I -	fracture line through the growth plate, separating epiphysis from metaphysis
II -	fracture line into the metaphysis
III -	separation of the epiphysis along the physis, with the fracture line passing through the epiphysis to the articular surface
IV -	fracture line crosses the physis, separating a peripheral fragment of bone that includes portions of epiphysis, physis, and metaphysis
V -	compression of the physis due to a severe axial load

Types III - V are potentially growth-limiting.

Section II: 50 Questions & Answers

Questions:

51. How do you treat Carbon Monoxide poisoning in pregnancy ?

52. How do you differentiate myoglobinuria from blood in the urine ?

53. How do you treat myoglobinuria ?

54. What is Conn's Syndrome ?

55. How does mannitol work ?

56. What two interleukins are produced by macrophages and monocytes ?

57. What are the two types of granules in platelets ?

58. How fast do you correct severe hyponatremia ?

59. What are the four classes of shock ?

60. How do you treat a Curling's Ulcer ?

61. Which class of shock do you begin to see a decrease in urine output ?

62. How do you estimate the size of an endotracheal tube in a child ?

63. What is SCIWORA ?

64. What are the features in Beck's Triad ?

65. How can you differentiate between tamponade and tension pneumothorax ?

66. How much hemoglobin do you need to look cyanotic ?

67. Where does the Internal Mammary Artery originate ?

68. What is the narrowest point in a child's airway ?

69. What is the first branch off of the subclavian artery ?

70. What metabolic disturbance may you see with Sulfamylon (and how does it work ?)

71. How do you treat "left-sided portal HTN" ?

72. What is the incubation period for *Clostridium tetani?*

73. In massive UGI bleeding, why is somatostatin safer to use compared to vasopressin ?

74. How do you treat an amebic liver abscess ?

75. How do you treat a Hydatid Cyst ?

76. What is phlegmasia cerulea dolens ?

77. What is the most common complication of stress gastritis ?

78. How do you treat a mutinodular goiter ?

79. What is the anatomical definition of "upper GI bleeding" ?

80. What is the false negative rate for a thyroid FNA?

81. What is the best diagnostic test for a suspected colovesical fistula ?

82. What is a Type III Gastric Ulcer ?

83. How do you calculate BMI ?

84. How do you treat Hashimoto's Thyroidistis ?

85. What is the Child's Classification ?

86. How do you treat a recurrent Phyllodes Tumor ?

87. What is a Chance Fracture ?

88. What are the risks for esophageal cancer ?

89. What must you consider in a patient with hypertension and a thyroid nodule ?

90. How do you treat a thyroid storm ?

91. How do you treat Malignant Hyperthermia ?

92. With a positive family history for malignant hyperthermia, how do you diagnose it in your patient ?

93. How do you treat the Fat Emboli Syndrome ?

94. What is ecthyma gangrenosum ?

95. How do you treat a duodenal hematoma ?

96. Why do you place a patient right-side up with air-embolism ?

97. What is the treatment of Von Willebrand's disease?

98. How much CSF is produced in one day ?

99. How do you treat DCIS ?

100. How do you treat LCIS ?

Answers:

51. Place on 100 % Oxygen and wait four-times longer than you would in a non-pregnant female – i.e. at least 4 hours (fetal Hb has a four-times higher affinity to carbon monoxide than adult Hb).

52. Both will be positive for blood on dipstick, but myoglobinuria will not have RBC's under the scope

53. Treatment of Myoglobinuria: fluid, fluid, fluid, and –
    a. Mannitol (25 – 50 g q 6 hrs)

    b. Bicarb Alkalinization (1 – 2 amps per liter of IVF)

    c. Fasciotomy, if indicated (the pt must be closely observed)

54. Conn's Syndrome: Primary Hyperaldosteronism

55. Two major effects of mannitol:
    a direct osmotic diuretic
    and a free radical scavenger

56. IL-1 and IL-6

57. Dense (energy proteins) and Alpha (procoagulants)

58. 1 mEq/hr, not to exceed 25 mEq's in 48 hour period; rare to use 3 % NaCl

59. Class I – IV

60. Curling's: stress ulcer associated with large-suface area burns

61. Class III

62. ET Tube: (Age / 4) + 4

63. Spinal Cord Injury Without Radiographic Abnormality
* always assume a c-spine injury !

64. JVD, Muffled Heart Tones, Hypotension

65. Tension PTX vs. Tamponade

66. You need at least 5 g of Hb to look cyanotic

67. Subclavian artery

68. Cricoid cartilage

69. The first branch off of the subclavian is the vertebral artery

70. Metabolic Acidosis secondary to carbonic anhydrase inhibition

71. Left-sided portal hypertension is due to splenic vein thrombosis (from pancreatitis, pancreatic cancer, retroperitoneal fibrosis...). The pt will present with a major gastric variceal bleed (not esophageal). The treatment is splenectomy, not TIPS.

72. 7 – 10 days

73. Vasopressin can cause coronary vasoconstriction

74. IV Flagyl for 3 weeks, and then, if necessary, percutaneous drainage

75. Echinococcal Cyst: Surgical treatment is effective in most cases. Be careful NOT to rupture the cyst because of the risk of implantation and anaphylaxis. Usually, attempts at aspiration and/or injection (i.e. hypertonic saline) are not very effective. Formalin and phenol have been injected in the past but this should be of historical interest only (because of the risk of damaging bile

ducts if a direct communication exists). The best way is to shell-out the cyst with a "rim" of hepatic tissue or by staying between the layers of endocyst and ectocyst. At times, hepatic lobectomy will be required. Albendazole is recommended afterwards to prevent recurrence.

76. Phlegmasia cerulean dolens: the most severe form of ileofemoral thrombosis. It is a severe obstruction of the venous outflow leading to arterial insuffiency, cyanosis, and eventual gangrene.

77. Bleeding; stress gastritis usually does not lead to perforation.

78. Subtotal thyroidectomy

79. Bleeding which occurs proximal to the ligament of Treitz

80. False Negative Rate of Thyroid FNA: Less than 6%

81. CT Scan

82. Type III Gastric Ulcer: a pre-pyloric ulcer

83. BMI = weight (kg) / height (m)^2

84. Treatment of Hashimoto's Thyroiditis:
    an autoimmune disease treated by suppressive
    doses of thyroid hormone (once the diagnosis has
    been established)

85. Child-Pugh Classification of functional status:

	A	**B**	**C**
Ascites	absent	slight-moderate	tense
Encephalopathy	none	grades I – II	III-IV
Serum Albumin	> 3.5	3.0 - 3.5	< 3.0
Serum Bilirubin	< 2.0	2.0 - 3.0	> 3.0
PT (above normal)	< 4	4 - 6	> 6

* Expected Mortality Rates:

A	~ 5%
B	~ 15%
C	~ 50%

86. Re-excison to negative margins.

    Axillary dissection, chemotherapy, and radiation
    are all unnecessary.

87. Chance Fx: a lumbar fracture associated with seat-
    belt injuries; strongly consider the presence of an
    associated small bowel injury

88. Risks of Esophageal Cancer:

> *Smoking*
> *Alcohol (?)*
> *Achalasia*
> *Celiac Sprue*
> *Plummer-Vinson*
> *Caustic Strictures*
> *Pickled / Cured Foods*
> *HPV Infection*
> *Malnutrition*
> *Obesity*
> *Barrett's Intestinal Metaplasia*

89. Pheochromocytoma

90. B-blocker (Inderal) and PTU

91. Dantrolene

92. Perform a muscle biopsy under local anesthesia; histology will be characteristic.

93. Treatment is supportive (oxygenation, ventilation, fluid support)

94. A green blister filled with *Pseudomonas* organisms

95. Observation with NGT decompression, NPO, and TPN for 2 weeks – far majority will resolve. If seen during an exploration for other reasons, then open evacuation

96. To keep the air in the right ventricle - you are trying to keep air from "locking" in the PA

97. Cryoprecipitate

98. About 500 cc's / day

99. WLE + Post-op Radiation

100.   Close follow-up and observation; pt is at higher risk of developing invasive ductal cancer

Section 3: 50 Questions & Answers

Questions:

101. Which one carries a better prognosis, EDH or SDH ?

102. When do you elevate table fractures of the skull? (and why ?)

103. What is the significance to "sulfur granules" ?

104. What is the most common skin manifestation in HIV patients ?

105. You're a surgeon…name 2 spirochetes ?

106. Which space-occupying lesion is the most common in HIV ?

107. Does endoscopic banding work for gastric varices ?

108. What is Grave's Disease ?

109. How do you treat duodenal atresia ?

110. How do you diagnose and treat malrotation ?

111. When would you want to keep a PDA open ?

112. What do you administer to close a PDA ?

113. Will Positive Pressure Ventilation, by itself, increase or decrease CVP ?

114. Where do you place a Greenfield filter for lower extremity DVT ?

115. What level corresponds radiographically to the renal veins ?

116. What are Ranson's Criteria at 48 hours ?

117. What chromosome is responsible for MEN-II ?

118. What is the primary effect of heparin ?

119. What is the clinical significance of a negative D-dimer ?

120. What is the normal SvO_2 ? (and what PO_2 does it correspond to ?)

121. What are the three reasons for a marginal ulcer ?

122. What is the most objective measure of a true compartment syndrome ?

123. What are the three zones of the neck ?

124. What is the maximal height you should raise the barium column when trying to reduce an intussception ?

125. What are the Class I antigens ? (and what cells are they found on ?)

126. What is Milroy's Disease ?

127. What does OKT3 target ?

128. What is the usual maximal-preservation time in UW solution for the following organs:
    ➢ Kidneys ?
    ➢ Pancreas ?
    ➢ Liver ?
    ➢ Heart / Lungs / Small Bowel ?

129. How do you repair ureteral transection ?

130. How do you treat CMV ?

131. What causes "dimpling" of the skin in breast cancer ?

132. What is the breast bud ?

133. How do you treat a Phylloides Tumor ?

134. What is Cushing's Syndrome ?

135. What is Paget's Disease of the breast ?

136. What defines Stage I breast cancer ?

137. What drug can be administered in an attempt to relieve a colonic pseudo-obstruction ?

138. How do you treat a Type IV Gastric Ulcer ?

139. Which form of Barret's esophagitis has malignant potential ?

140. How do you treat Stage II breast cancer ?

141. How do you diagnose and treat inflammatory breast cancer ?

142. What causes early-dumping ? (how do you treat it ?)

143. What causes late-dumping ? (how do you treat it?)

144. What is the Nigro Protocol ?

145. How do you treat an anal melanoma ?

146. How do you treat a chronic anal fissure ?

147. How do you calculate the RQ ?

148. When do you proceed with a lymph node dissection, in melanoma ?

149. How do you treat a melanoma on the anterior face ?

150. How do you treat a melanoma on the scalp or ear ?

Answers:

101.   EDH – there is less underlying parenchymal injury than seen in SDH

102.   When the depression is greater than 1 cm – this decreases the risk of seizures

103.   Actinomycosis – remember, this is a bacterial infection *(treat with high-dose PCN)*

104.   Molluscum contagiosum

105.   2 spirochetes:

    1.) *Borrelia* (Lyme disease, relapsing fever)
    Tx with ceftriaxone

    2.) *Treponema* (Syphilis)
    Tx with PCN

106.   Toxoplasmosis

107.   No, banding only works for esophageal varices. With gastric varices, and true portal hypertension, you will likely require TIPS

108.   Hyperthyroidism due to the formation of an autoimmune antibody directed against the TSH receptor; treatment of choice is radioactive ablation (I 131)

109.   Duodenal atresia:
        side-to-side duodenoduodenostomy with a decompressive g-tube

110.   Lower GI – look for the cecum in the LUQ

111.   Coarctation of the aorta; you keep the PDA open by administering prostaglandin

112.   Indomethacin

113.   Positive pressure increases CVP

114.   Below the renal veins (if there is thrombosis of the filter, you do no want to occlude the renals)

115.   L2

116.   Ranson's Criteria of severity:

Admission:
Age > 55   0 - 2 = 2% mortality
WBC > 16,000
Glucose > 200   3 – 4 = 15% mortality
LDH > 350
SGOT > 250   5 – 6 = 40% mortality

At 48 hours:
Hct fall > 10%   > 7 = 100% mort.
BUN rise > 8
Serum Ca < 8
Arterial PO^2 < 60
Base Deficit > 4
Fluid Sequestration > 6 L

117.   Chromosome # 10

118.   Stimulates Anti-thrombin III

119.   A negative d-dimer effectively rules-out a pulmonary embolus

120.   75 (40)

121.   Incomplete vagotomy, incomplete antrectomy, Z-E Syndrome

122.   Intracompartmental pressures > 30 mmHg (indication for urgent fasciotomy)

123. Zone I: from the clavicles to cricoid
Zone II: from cricoid to the mandibular angle
Zone III: from the mandibular angle to the
base of the skull

124. 3 feet

125. A, B – found on all nucleated cells

126. Milroy's: a chronic hereditary lymphedema
with onset at or near birth (in a few patients it
does not develop until after the age of 35,
i.e."lymphedema tarda"). It is caused by a
developmental abnormality of the lymphatics

127. The CD3 receptor

128. kidneys – 48 hrs; pancreas – 24 hrs; liver – 12
hrs; heart, lung, small bowel – 8 hrs

129. There are several ways to repair an accidental
transection; the one I prefer is an interrupted,
primary repair using 5-0 dacron sutures over a 6fr.
Double-J silastic stent.

The stent is removed via cytsocopy 6 weeks after
the repair. I always leave a drain behind (but some
do not).

130. Gancyclovir

131. Involvement of Cooper's Ligaments (not lymphatic invasion or "skin edema")

132. The breast bud is a normal, developmental structure seen at the onset of puberty. It should never be biopsied!

133. A Phyllodes tumor is an uncommon stromal lesion consisting of both epithelial and mesenchymal cells. The far majority (> 90 %) are completely benign and related to fibroadenoma. Treatment is via wide local excision to negative margins and there is no role for axillary dissection or adjuvant therapy.

134. Cushing's Syndrome is the state of hypercortisolism. Unfortunately, the term has been used carelessly in the past which has led to confusion regarding the underlying disease process.

   Primary Hypercortisolism (the real, "Cushing's syndrome", i.e. related to a primary disease within the adrenal gland), is seen with an adrenal tumor.

   Cushing's Disease is due to a central process (usually a pituitary tumor) which release an excess of ACTH and thus produces a Secondary Hypercortisolism.

135.   Paget's disease of the breast is Invasive Ductal Carcinoma involving the nipple-areola complex; a palpable mass may or may not be present. It is treated by Modified Radical Mastectomy.

136.   Stage I Breast Cancer: T1, No, Mo (a T1 lesion is less than 2 cm in total diameter). Treat with Breast-conserving therapy !

137.   Neostigmine 2 mg IV over 5 minutes with EKG monitoring

    pt must not have peritoneal signs or a true volvulus

    over 90 % effective

    dose may be repeated in 3 hrs. if necessary

    may cause symptomatic bradycardia in 20 % of pts.
    (treated with Atropine)

138.   Treatment of a Type IV Gastric Ulcer: Excision. (maintaining the GE Junction is preferred if anatomically possible)

139.   Intestinal Metaplasia

140.   Treatment of a Stage II Breast CA: Breast-
        conserving therapy (i.e. lumpectomy, XRT, &
        sentinel-node biopsy). At present, little role of
        MRM.

141.   Treatment of Inflammatory Breast CA:

        Biopsy the lesion.

        Rule out metastases with mammography,
        bone scans and a CT scan of the chest,
        abdomen, brain (and axilla ?).

        Begin neoadjuvant therapy with
        FAC/CAFV/CMF.

        After an initial course (4 - 6 weeks), complete
        the mastectomy and axillary dissection
        followed by radiation therapy and adjuvant
        chemotherapy.

        If no response is obtained with chemotherapy
        initially, then proceed with radiation therapy.

        Proceed with mastectomy if possible after
        radiation therapy and follow with adjuvant
        chemotherapy.

        Overall prognosis is poor with a median
        survival of 31 months

142.   Early dumping : Hyperosmolar Load

143.   Late dumping: Inappropriate Insulin
Response

144.   The Nigro Protocol – given for all biopsy-
proven anal carcinoma *(except melanoma)*

5-FU, 1000 mg IV qd for the first 3 days of
therapy

200 rads external beam radiation, M – F for 5 wks

Last 3 days of treatment, 5-FU, 1000 mg IV qd

Re-examine the pt in 2 weeks

If no visible tumor remaining, do a biopsy of the
area

If biopsy is negative, treatment is finished and pt
undergoes close follow-up
If biopsy is positive, Give 1000 Rads of radiation
for a total of 6,000 then re-biopsy

If gross tumor remains after the 5000 Rads, then
APR

If there is clinically-positive nodes, then perform a
superficial groin dissection (you should never
irradiate a groin)

145.   Wide local excision

146.   Botox injection

147. $RQ = CO_2$ Produced / O_2 Consumed

148.   When the melanoma is "Intermediate Thickness", 1 – 4 mm

149.   Anterior face Melanoma:

Wide local excision with Superficial Parotidectomy and Modified Radical Neck Dissection

150.   Wide Local Excision *(may require plastic reconstruction after excision)*

Section 4: 50 Questions & Answers

Questions:

151. What is the most common primary liver tumor?

152. How do you calculate: MAP ?
                                 CO ?
                                 SVR ?

153. How do you treat a GSW to the rectum ?

154. Where does the aorta perforate in a "jumper"
      that hits 'feet-first' ?

155. Why would a young, healthy woman present to
      the ED with sudden-onset hypotension ?

156. What will improve the appetite in HIV patients
      or in chronic-cancer patients ?

157. How do you treat an elevated bleeding time ?

158. How do you treat Mobitz-type II ?

159. How do you treat peaked T waves ?

160. What three things do you need to have 'ARDS'?

161. What is the first clinical sign of hypermagnesemia ?

162. What is the most common cause of hypoxemia in a surgical patient ?

163. How do you manage "follicular hyperplasic" on a thyroid FNA ?

164. What can a posterior dislocation of the clavicle cause ? (how do you treat it ?)

165. What level is the tracheal bifurcation at ?

166. What is the pulmonary ligament ?

167. Which intercostal space is the widest ?

168. In cancer, when do you see an "onion-skin appearance"?

169. In cancer, when do you see a "sunbusrt-appearance"?

170. How do you calculate an Anion Gap ?

171. What causes a normal-AG acidosis ?

172. What is the best operation to perform for
      secondary hyperparathyroidism ?

173. What is phlegmasia alba dolens ?

174. What is the clinical half-life:

      Albumin ?
      Transferrin ?
      Prealbumin ?
      Retinol Binding Protein ?

175. What is Mondor's Disease ?

176. What is the meaning of an RQ of 0.7 ?

177. How do you treat "Gallbladder Ca" found by
      the pathologist following a lap chole ?

178. What is the significance of UUN ?

179. What is the mortality rate of an aspiration
      episode ?

180. What is the most common nosocomial
      infection?

181. What are the Vitamin K-dependent factors ?

182. Why does "purified-Factor VIII" not work for Von Willebrand's disease ?

183. How do you treat a low-grade MALT ?

184. What is a Zenker's Diverticulum ?

185. How do you treat a sigmoid volvulus ?

186. When do you see "Reed-Sternberg Cells" ?

187. Which anal cancers are related to human papilloma virus?

188. How do you diagnose a pheochromocytoma ?

189. How do you treat an acute, severe bleeding episode in a patient with known ITP ?

190. What is the most common location for an accessory spleen ?

191. What other conditions should you consider in a patient with SBO ?

192. How do you treat a cystadenocarcinoma of the appendix?

193. What valvular disease do you see in patients with the carcinoid syndrome ?

194. What is a Monteggia fracture ?

195. What is Phlegmasia alba dolens ?

196. How do you treat a 4 cm villous adenoma of the descending colon ?

197. What is the treatment for a benign-appearing gastric ulcer along the lesser curve ?

198. How do you treat a subclavian vein thrombosis secondary to central line placement ?

199. What are the two classic signs of arterial insuffiency ?

200. What is the most commonly-seen anatomy in popliteal artery syndrome ?

Answers:

151.   Hemangioma

152.   MAP = [(SBP - DBP) / 3] + DBP

CO = HR x SV

SVR = (MAP – CVP / CO) x 80 dynes-cm –5

153.   Presacral drainage ("u"-incision), with a diverting colostomy

154.   It tears at the aortic root, not at the ligamentum arteriosum

* also "common" in jumpers is renal artery avulsion

155.   Ectopic
Bleeding hepatoma
Ruptured splenic artery aneurysm

156.   Megace

157.   DDAVP, 0.3 units/kg – can be given twice in succession

158. Pacemaker

159. Peaked T waves = Hypercalcemia

 a. First, protect the myocardium: Calcium

 b. Second, 1 amp D50

 c. Third, administer insulin

 d. Fourth – must decrease the total body calcium

160. ARDS – 3 criteria:

 a. $PaO_2 / FiO_2 < 200$
 b. Bilateral infiltrates on CXR
 c. No evidence of CHF (Pw < 18)

161. Loss of Deep Tendon Reflexes

162. V-Q Mismatch

163. Thyroid Lobectomy with Isthmusectomy; if frozen section or permanent histology reveals true follicular carcinoma proceed with total thyroidectomy

164.   Tracheal Compression with airway
        compromise; treated by surgical reduction

165.   T4

166.   The pulmonary ligament is a reflection of the
        visceral pleura

167.   The 3rd intercostals space

168.   "Onion-skin" = Ewing's Sarcoma

169.   "Sunburst Appearance" = Osteogenic
        Sarcoma

170. $AG = (Na^+ + K^+) - (Cl^- + HCO_3^-)$

171.   Normal AG Acidosis
        Diarrhea
        Fistulas
        Renal Tubular Acidosis

172.   Kidney Transplant

173.   Phelgmasia alba dolens: a variant of
        ileofemoral thrombosis characterized by arterial
        spasm and a pale, cool leg with diminished pulses
        (treated via heparinization)

174.   Half-Life:

Albumin   -   18 days
Transferrin   -   8 days
Prealbumin   -   3 days
Retinol Binding Protein   -   12 hrs

175.   Mondor's Disease: a localized thrombophlebitis of the anterolateral chest wall

176.   RQ = 0.7; this means that fats are being utilized as the primary fuel source

177.   Gallbladder Ca on the path report: reoperation for wedge resection of the liver bed plus regional lymhadenectomy

178.   UUN – urine urea nitrogen, a guide to nitrogen balance

UUN   =   N2 Intake   -   N2 Ouput
UUN   =   (G protein/6.25)   -   (UUN + 4)

179.   Mortality approaches 50%

180.   UTI

181.   II, VII, IX, and X

182.   "Purified Factor VIII" does not contain VonWillebrand's Factor – which is the deficiency in Von Willebrand's disease

183.   Treat the associated *H. pylori* !

184.   Zenker's Diverticulum:
a paryngoesophageal pulsion diverticulum that arises in the posterior midline of the neck - just above the cricopharyngeus muscle and below the inferior constrictor (surgical therapy is the treatment of choice - excision with myotomy of the cricopharyngeal muscle)

185.   Sigmoid Volvulus: colonoscopic decompression

186.   Reed-Sternberg Cells = "owl-eye cells" = Hodgkin's lymphoma

187.   All anal cancers are associated with Human Papilloma Virus

188.   Pheo = Urinary Metanephrines

189.   Gamma-globulin

190.   Splenic hilum

191.   Small Bowel Obstruction: *(after adhesions from previous surgery)*

   a. Hernias
   b. Crohn's disease
   c. Carcinoid

192.   Right hemicolectomy, and consider taking out both ovaries (especially in a post-menopausal female; they are more likely to develop ovarian cancer)

193.   Tricuspid Insuffiency

194.   The "night-stick fracture": a common story is that of a burglar being hit by a police night-stick; the burglar brings his arm up to protect his face and sustains an ulnar fracture – commonly associated with a dislocated radial head…. get a lateral elbow film to rule-this out

195.   Phlegmasia alba dolens: "milk leg" "white leg"

   caused by extension of a DVT into the iliac system

   this is the first stage before the syndrome evolves into "phlegmasia cerulea dolens" (blue leg)

196.   Segmental colectomy with primary reanastamosis

197.   Treatment of a gastric ulcer: *consider resecting all gastric ulcers to rule-out CA*

Medical Management: Anti-secretory Agent (Proton Pump Inhibitor)

Antibiotics against H. pylori

D/C all Nsaid's & Cox II inhibitors

Indications for Surgery:	Biopsy positive or suspicious for malignancy
	Large ulcer *(especially if it is located along the greater curve)*
	Failure to heal with medical management after 3 months

198.   Remove the central line and heparinize the pt.

199.   Elevation pallor & Dependent rubor

200.   The most commonly seen abnormality leading to popliteal entrapment is an artery that runs medial to the medial head of the gastrocnemius

Section 5: 50 Questions & Answers

Questions:

201. How do you treat DCIS ?

202. How do you treat an incidentally-found ovarian/adnexal mass ?

203. How do you treat a tubo-ovarian abscess ?

204. How does IABP (intra-aortic balloon pump) improve hemodynamics ?

205. When is IABP contraindicated ?

206. What syndrome includes a necrloytic migratory erythema ?

207. How do you confirm the diagnosis of carcinoid syndrome ?

208. What criteria meet "critical" aortic stenosis ?

209. What criteria meet "critical" mitral stenosis ?

210. What is the most common cause of a solid renal mass in an adult ?

211. How do you treat an intra-caval renal cell cancer?

212. How do you treat a testicular mass ?

213. What are the serum markers in testicular cancer?

214. What is the BIRADS Classification ?

215. What is the first test for a palpable breast mass ?

216. What is the most effective treatment for an aspiration episode ?

217. How do you treat clear, serous discharge from a single duct in the female breast ?

218. What is the most common palpable breast mass in a pregnant female ?

219. What is the operative approach to a thoracic duct leak ?

220. What causes most bloody nipple discharge ?

221. What chromosome is responsible for Gardner's syndrome ?

222. What are the "Amsterdam Criteria" ?

223. When do you see a bird's beak esophagus ?

224. What is the most common cause of lower GI bleeding ?

225. What is the most common cause of Massive lower GI bleeding ?

226. What is the most common cause of Massive lower GI bleeding in patients > age 70 ?

227. How do you treat an infected urachal cyst ?

228. What level differentiates colon cancer from rectal cancer ?

229. How do you approach a BIRADS 0 classification ?

230. What is a Stage III colon cancer ?

231. When do you administer preoperative neoadjuvant therapy for esophageal cancer ?

232. Where is iron absorbed ?

233. What is the most common cause of Portal HTN in the United States ?

234. What is the Budd-Chiari Syndrome ?

235. What is the best way to prevent a first bleed in a portal HTN patient ?

236. What is the preferred treatment of Ascites ?

237. What is the preferred treatment for Grave's Disease ?

238. How do you treat a 3 cm. Appendiceal Carcinoid ?

239. What are the two main risk factors for Papillary Thyroid CA ?

240. How does follicular thyroid cancer spread ?

241. What do C-cells produce ?

242. What is the origin of the Superior Thyroid Artery ?

243. How do you treat a duodenal diverticulum ?

244. What is the most common manifestation of the Carcinoid Syndrome ?

245. What are 3 extra-colonic manifestations associated with Ulcerative Colitis ?

246. What is the half-life of Parathyroid Hormone ?

247. What is the best diagnostic screen for a "lost parathyroid" ?

248. What is the most common cause of a "cushing's picture" ?

249. What is the most common cause of primary hyperparathyroidism ?

250. How do you treat a 100 % occlusion of the internal carotid artery ?

Answers:

201. DCIS: wide local excision to negative
margins, followed by XRT to the
ipsilateral breast

202. The "Incidental Ovarian Mass"

    a. First, always perform the operation
that you went there to perform
    b. Remember, you can always come back
    c. Then, describe fully what you see
i.e. peritoneal studding, omental
caking...

- never do a wedge
biopsy of the mass or
ovary
- never do a TAH-BSO,
at the time of initial
discovery

203. Antibiotics, antibiotics, antibiotics....

When you find a tubo-ovarian abscess, you
are likely exploring for suspected appendicitis;
perform the appendectomy and describe the
relevant findings. Unless the ovary is necrotic
or gangrenous, do not proceed with resection
(especially in the pre-menopausal female). If
the abscess progresses or begins to lead to
septic complications, you can always go back
and resect.

204. 2 effects of IABP:
     a. Increases coronary blood flow
     b. decreases afterload

205. IABP is contraindicated in:
     a. Aortic regurgitation
     b. Lower limb ischemia

206. Glucagonoma

207. Carcinoid Diagnosis: Check Urinary 5-HIAA level

208. Critical aortic stenosis: Area < 1 cm^2
                                    $P > 50$ mmHg

209. Critical mitral stenosis: Area < 1.5 cm^2
                                    $P > 15$ mmHg

210. Renal Cell CA

211. Resection; intracaval spread does not preclude a full and complete resection, i.e. a radical nephrectomy without previous biosy.

212. A testicular mass is cancer till proven otherwise and should be treated with an inguinal orchiectomy. Do not violate the median raphe or perform a scrotal biopsy.

213. Serum markers in testicular cancer: *AFP*
                                                     B-HCG
                                                     LDH

214. BIRADS Classification:

     "0"   -   inadequate mammogram

     "I"   -   normal mammogram

     "II"   -   radiographic abnormality
                           present, likely benign

     "III" -   undetermined lesion, low
                           suspicion for carcinoma

     "IV" -   suspicious lesion present

     "V"   -   malignancy strongly suspected
                           (i.e. a solid mass with calcifications)

215. FNA

216. Aggressive suctioning – consider endotracheal intubation and formal bronchoscopy

217. Ductogram followed by complete ductal excision

218. Lactating adenoma

219. Right Thoracoctomy – with ligation of the duct just above the diaphragm *(VATS if available)*

220. Papilloma

221. Chromosome 5q

222. Amsterdam Criteria: the Lynch Syndrome

> 3 relatives
> in 2 or more generations
> where at least 1 is a first-degree relative

223. Achalasia

224. Colonic neoplasia

225. Diverticulosis

226. A-V Malformations

227. Antibiotics, followed by complete excision (including the associated cuff of bladder)

228. 12 cm. from the dentate line – above is condidered "colon" & below is "rectum"

229. You must repeat the mammogram, and may require cone-views

230. Duke's Colon Ca:

    A -   Limited to the Bowel Wall

    B -   Extension through the Bowel Wall with Negative Nodes

    C -   Regional Node Metastasis

    Duke's Modification:
    C_1 -   Regional Node Metastasis
    C_2 -   Node Involvement at the Point of Vessel Ligation

231. Stage II or Stage III Esophageal CA

232. Duodenum

233. Alcoholic cirrhosis

234. Budd-Chiari Syndrome:

    hepatic vein thrombosis leading to post-sinusoidal portal hypertension

235. Beta-blockade is the only proven method to prevent a FIRST bleed

236. Medical management:

> fluid & salt restriction
> spironolactone
>
> surgery carries a minimal role in the direct
> treatment of ascites

237. I^{131} Ablation, followed by supplemental replacement

238. Right hemicolectomy with ileocolic anastamosis, and remember to take the regional nodes.

239. Risk Factors – Papillary CA:
> Childhood exposure to Radiation
> Positive family history

240. Follicular cancer does not spread through the lymphatics; it spreads hematogenously to bone and lung

241. Calcitonin

242. The external carotid artery

243. Resect the diverticulum

244. Diarrhea

245. Erythema nodosum, erythema multiforme, & pyoderma gangrensum (just to name a few)

246. 8 minutes, this is why on-table PTH levels are helpful in parathyroid surgery

247. Sestamibi scan

248. Exogenous steroid use

249. A single adenoma

250. 100% occlusion. Place on ASA qd and follow the contralateral carotid with surveillance duplex sreening

Section 6: A Bonus - 25 Questions & Answers

What is the Diagnosis ?

251.   What is the diagnosis:
        a child presents with unilateral ptosis?

252.   What is the diagnosis:
        C-spine film with a 25 % over-ride?

253.   What is the diagnosis:
        C-spine film with a 50 % over-ride?

254.   What is the diagnosis:
        a patient presents with bilateral pinpoint
        pupils ?

255.   What is the diagnosis:
        'brownish-fluid leaking from a wound, with
        Gm + Rods?

256.   What is the diagnosis:
        a patient steps on a nail and develops
        subsequent infection?

257.   What is the diagnosis:
        a trauma patient has a positive Sudan's stain?

258.   What is the diagnosis:
       a patient develops nuchal rigidity just after
       intubation?

259.   What is the diagnosis:
       upper GI reveals a "stack of coins"?

260.   What is the diagnosis:
       a dropping fluid level on CXR, s/p
       pneumonectomy?

261.   What is the diagnosis:
       esophageal manometry demonstrates an
       elevated resting LES pressure with non-
       relaxation during swallowing ?

262.   What is the diagnosis:
       pediatric patient with massive UGI bleeding?

263.   What is the diagnosis:
       young male with syncopal episode, BP 60/30,
       HR 40?

264.   What is the diagnosis:
       barium swallow demonstrates a "corkscrew
       esophagus"?

265.   What is the diagnosis:
       plain radiograph with "double bubble"
       appearance?

266. What is the diagnosis:
persistent hypocalcemia despite multiple bolus
replacements?

267. What is the diagnosis:
RQ > 1.1?

268. What is the diagnosis:
sudden chest pain during esophageal dilation?

269. What is the diagnosis:
a positive osmotic fragility test?

270. What is the diagnosis:
amyloid deposition on fine needle aspirate of
a thyroid nodule ?

271. What is the diagnosis:
scimitar sign on angiographic evaluation?

272. What is the diagnosis:
palpable neck mass with hypercalcemia?

273. What is the diagnosis:
elevated airway pressures with decreased urine
output?

274.　What is the diagnosis:
　　　8 wk. old male infant with projectile vomiting
　　　and dehydration?

275.　What is the diagnosis:
　　　26 yr. old pregnant female with LUQ "egg-
　　　shell calcifications"?

Answers:

251. Myasthenia gravis – thymoma

252. Unilateral locked facet

253. Bilateral locked facet

254. Pontine hemorrhage

255. *Clostridium perfringens*

256. *Psuedomonas*

257. Fat emboli syndrome

258. Malignant hyperthermia

259. Duodenal hematoma

260. Bronchpleural fistula

261. Achalasia

262. Portal vein thrombosis

263. Vasovagal episode

264. Diffuse Esophageal spasm

265. Duodenal atresia

266. Hypomagnesemia

267. Over-feeding

268. Rule-out MI, likely an esophageal perforation

269. Hereditary spherocytosis

270. Medullary thyroid cancer

271. Popliteal cystic disease

272. Parathyroid cancer

273. Abdominal compartment syndrome

274. Pyloric stenosis

275. Splenic artery aneurysm

Review Topics

A. Acid Base Disorders

General Concepts

Normal blood pH is 7.40 (7.36 – 7.44), which corresponds to a [H+] of 40 nEq/L (44-36).

Systemic arterial pH is maintained by complex buffering mechanisms as well as renal and respiratory compensatory responses.

The kidneys regulate HCO_3^- by the following mechanisms:

> Reabsorption of filtered HCO_3^-
> Formation of titrable acid
> Excretion of NH_4^+ in the urine

Acidemia: serum pH < 7.36
Alkalemia: serum pH > 7.44

Acidosis: pathophysiologic processes, which favor development of acidemia

Alkalosis: pathophysiologic processes, which favor development of alkalemia

Buffer: A substance, which can absorb or donate H+ ions in order to mitigate changes pH.

$$H_2CO_3^- \leftrightarrow H^+ + HCO_3^- \leftrightarrow H_2O + CO_2$$

* Remember: [H+] ion concentration and pH are inversely related.

Henderson-Hasselbalch equation:

$$pH = pK + \log \frac{(HCO3^-)}{(PaCO2)} \qquad pK = 6.1$$

Kassirer-Bleich equation:

$$H+ = 24 \times PCO2/HCO3^-$$

Reflects how the acidity of blood is determined by the relative availability of acid and alkali, i.e. $HCO3^-$, $PaCO2$. Stresses how H+ ion concentration is determined by the ratio of $PCO2/HCO3$, rather than the absolute value of either value alone.

Remember:
Metabolic Acidosis/Alkalosis = disturbances of blood bicarbonate

Respiratory Acidosis/Alkalosis = disturbances of PaCO2

Metabolic Acidosis

Anion Gap: $Na+ - (Cl^- + HCO3^-)$

(represents unmeasured anions in plasma, normally 10-12 mmol/L)

Elevated AG	Decreased AG	Normal AG *(hyperchloremic)*
Ethylene glycol	Hypercalcemia	Diarrhea
Lactic acid	Hypermagnesemia	RTA
Methanol	Hyperkalemia	Acetazolamide
Paraldehyde	Hypoalbuminemia	Diversions (ureteral)
ASA	Paraproteinemia	Renal failure
Renal failure	Lithium toxicity	HCL administration

Ketoacidosis

<u>Compensation:</u>

Winter's formula: $PaCO2 = 1.5 \times HCO3^- + 8 \ (+/-2)$

(PaCO2 = last 2 digits of pH…chronic metabolic acidosis)

<u>Treatment:</u>

Should be directed at the underlying cause

Bicarbonate therapy can be considered with severe acidosis with physiologic compromise:

Bicarbonate deficit(mEq) =
$LBW \times 0.5 \times (Desired \ HCO3^- - Actual \ HCO3^-)$

Osmolal Gap: Measured OSM – Calculated OSM

Calculated Osmolality:

$2 \times Na + Glc/18 + BUN/2.8 + ETOH/4.6$

<u>Elevated OG (> 10 mOsm/L):</u>

Methanol
Ethylene glycol
Paraldehyde
ETOH ketoacidosis
Isopropyl alcohol

Mannitol
Metabolic Alkalosis

Cl⁻ responsive (Ucl <20)		Cl⁻ resistant (Ucl > 30)
GI:	NG suction	Primary mineralocorticoid excess
	Vomiting/diarrhea	Primary aldosteronism
	Laxative abuse	Cushing's syndrome
	Villous adenoma	
	Licorice	
Renal:	Diuretics	Alkali load
	Post hypercapnea	Citrate (transfusions)
	Refeeding alkalosis	Acetate (TPN)
	Cystic fibrosis (sweat)	Bartter's syndrome
	Severe hypokalemia/-magnesemia	

Compensation:

$PaCO2 = 0.9 \times HCO3^- + 9$

Treatment:

Acetazolamide (Diamox): 250 -375 mg po qd-bid

HCl infusion:
       0.1-0.2 N @ < 0.2 mEq/hour via central line

HCL (mmol) = (LBW x 0.5) x Act HCO3- desired HCO3)

Hemodialysis: severe alkalosis with cardiac/renal dysfunction

Respiratory acidosis

CNS:
Sedatives, morphine, anesthetics
Trauma, Stroke
Infection

NM Disorders:
Myopathies (MD, K+ depletion)
Neuropathies (GB, polio)

Acute-Chronic Lung disease
COPD
PNA, pulmonary edema
ARDS
Acute obstruction (aspiration, tumor, spasm)
Obesity
Pneumothorax
Pleural effusion
Kyphoscoliosis
Scleroderma
Crush injury
Mechanical ventilation
Cardiopulmonary arrest

Compensation:

Acute: $HCO3^-$ increases by 1 mmol/L for
            each 10 mm Hg increase in PaCO2

Chronic: $HCO3^-$ increases by 4 mmol/L for
            each 10 mm Hg increase in PaCO2

Respiratory alkalosis

Anxiety, Pain
CNS Disorders (CVA, tumor, infection)
Lung Disease:
      Restrictive disorders
      Pulmonary embolus
      PNA
Sepsis, fever
Hyperthryoidism
Hypoxia
Hepatic insufficiency
Pregnancy
Salicylates, Catecholamines
Mechanical ventilation

Compensation:

Acute: HCO_3^- decreases by 2 mmol/L for each 10 mm Hg decrease in $PaCO_2$

Chronic: HCO_3^- decreases by 5-7 mmol/L for each 10 mm Hg decrease in $PaCO_2$

Delta Gap:

Identifies triple acid base disorders
Δ gap = Δ AG = Δ HCO3

ΔAG/ΔHCO3:	≤ 1	> 1
	Non AG acidosis	Metabolic alkalosis + AG acidosis
	DKA	Lactic acidosis

Chronic renal failure

Summary of Acid Base Compensatory Responses

Primary disorder	Primary Expected	Response
Metabolic Acidosis	↓ HCO_3- ↓ $PaCO_2$	$PCO_2 = 1.5$ x $HCO_3 + 8$ (+/-2)

$PaCO_2$ = last 2 digits of pH
$PaCO_2$ ↓ 1.25mm Hg ~ 1 mmol/L ↓ HCO_3

Metabolic Alkalosis	↑ HCO_3^- ↑ $PaCO_2$	$PaCO_2 = 0.9$ x $HCO_3 + 9$

$PaCO_2 = HCO_3 + 15$
$PaCO_2$ ↑ 6 mm Hg ~ 10 mmol/L ↑ HCO_3

Respiratory Acidosis	↑ $PaCO_2$ ↓ HCO_3^-	Acute: HCO_3 ↑ 1 mmol/L ~ 10 mmHg ↑ $PaCO_2$
		Chronic: HCO_3 ↑ 4 mmol/L ~ 10 mm Hg ↑ $PaCO_2$

Respiratory Alkalosis	↓ $PaCO_2$ ↑ HCO_3^-	Acute: HCO_3^- ↓2mmol/L ~ 10 mm Hg ↓ $PaCO_2$
		Chronic: HCO_3^- ↓5mmol/L

PaCO2

B. Hemodynamics

Before discussing basic hemodynamics, we should remind ourselves of the systemic circuit:
1. Cardiac Anatomy
2. Circulatory Pathways

Cardiac Anatomy

The Heart: 2 Separate Volume Pumps!
- **RA & RV** - Low Pressure "Bellows"
- **LA & LV** - High Pressure "Drive"

the in-series nature of these two systems implies that the output of the Right Heart becomes the input of the Left Heart, and therefore, the output of the Left Heart becomes the input of the Right Heart

1. Flow via Series
2. Demonstrated by William Harvey, 1628

- The Heart is a muscular organ enclosed in a fibrous sac (the *Pericardium)*
- Cardiac Muscle is termed the *Myocardium*
- The inner surface of the myocardium (the one icontact with the blood) is lined by a thin layer of *Endothelium*
- The Heart is divided into Right & Left Halves
  - Each consisting of an atrium & ventricle
  - Separated by the Atrioventricular Valves: Tricuspid
    Mitral

- Openings of the RV into the Pulmonary Trunk & the LV into the Aorta are also regulated by Valves:
Pulmonic
      Aortic

  1. Valve Function is a **Passive Process**
  2. Function of Papillary Muscles

Desaturated Blood returns from the Systemic Vessels via **the SVC & IVC**

  - Is displaced passively (and actively with atrial contraction) through the Tricuspid Valve - into the Right Ventricle.

  - Contraction of the RV ejects this volume through the Pulmonic Valve and into the Low-Pressure Pulmonary Artery, (PAP 5 - 12) then through the associated end-capillaries where gas-exchange occurs

Saturated Blood is then returned to the Left Atrium via the Pulmonary Veins
- In the LA, the blood is displaced to the LV **(15 - 20 % Atrial "Kick")**

- With LV Contraction, blood is forced through the aortic valve into the high-pressure aorta **(SBP 120 - 160)** thus perfusing the brain, kidneys, abdominal viscera, and extremities

Myocardial Perfusion
occurs primarily during Diastole

Myocardial Blood Flow:
1. Flow is provided by the Right & Left Coronary Arteries which are the first branches of the aorta, arising from the **Sinuses of Valsalva**

2. RCA - supplies the RV Wall, Sinus Node, and AV Node in 90 % of pts, the RCA terminates as the Posterior Descending Artery (Right Coronary Dominance)

3. The Left Main Coronary gives rise to both LAD & Circumflex

4. The LAD is usually the **largest** of all coronary arteries and supplies the anterior / apical LV, the majority of the IV Septum, and the left side of the RV

5. The Circumflex supplies the lateral LV and in 10 % of pts provides the Posterior Descending Coronary (Left Coronary Dominance)

6. Venous Drainage of the Heart
* Occurs mainly via the **Coronary Sinus** (into the RA).

Anterior Cardiac Veins
also: Thebesian Channels
          Sinusoidal Paths

Total Coronary Flow:
0.7 - 0.9 ml/min/g myocardium

Myocyte Contraction

Chemical Energy................Mechanical Energy
(Oxygen & Substrate)   *(Pressure & Flow)*

at the cellular level, electrical depolarization of the
myocardial cell membrane allows ionized calcium flux
into the cytoplasm - leading to hydrolysis of ATP by
Myosin.

This leads to a conformational change in the **Actin-
Myosin Cross Bridge** producing sliding of myosin
filaments relative to actin & overall shortening of the
sarcomere **[Sliding Filament Theory]**

* Calcium is then removed from the cell by **Active
Transport** in the Sarcoplasmic Reticulum - allowing
Relaxation, while ATP is regenerated by Metabolic
Processes

Over the physiologic range of sarcomere length (1.6 -
2.0 um), the amount of metabolic energy converted to
mechanical work is **dependent** on the available
Surface Area of Cross-Bridge Interactions

* Work is **directly proportional** to End-Diastolic
Sarcomere Length

This **"Length Dependency"** is the fundamental
basis for the **Frank-Starling Law**

- Otto Frank, 1885 *(Frog Heart Preparations)*

"the output of a normal heart is influenced primarily by the volume of blood in the ventricle at the end of diastole"

- Ernest Starling, 1914
  (extended this basic principle to mammalian hearts)

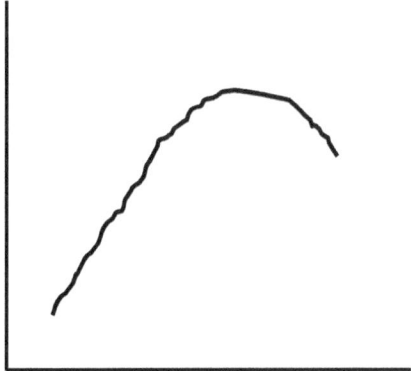

- Relationship: **EDV to SP**

- The Steep Ascending Portion of the Curve ! this area indicates the ***importance of PreLoad*** (i.e. Volume) for augmenting Output

- The **"Descending Limb"**
  - As EDV becomes Excessive, Pressure begins to Fall
  - WHY?
  - Is it Clinically Significant?

Cardiac Output: CO = HR x SV

"the amount of blood pumped by the heart per unit time"

Normal C.O. : 3.5 - 8.5 L/min

Manipulation of the factors can lead to augmentation of CO at the lowest possible energy cost

Determinants of Cardiac Performance & Output

Preload: EDV *(the load that stretches a muscle prior to contraction)*

Afterload: SVR *(the load that must be moved during muscle contraction)*

Contractility: the velocity of muscle shortening at a constant preload and afterload

Compliance: the length that a muscle is stretched by a given preload…….Determined by the inherent **Elasticity**

Heart Rate: several effects on overall Cardiac Function
* Tachycardia/Bradycardia

Preload
- At the cellular level, Preload is defined as end-diastolic sarcomere length which is linearly related to EDV.

- **Problem:** We can not measure Ventricular Volume in the Clinical Setting (rather impractical)

- LVEDP represents the Distending Pressure (the **Filling Pressure**) of the Ventricle and can be used as an index of EDV

-
- However, this Relationship is Exponential, NOT Linear

-
- In Normal Hearts, **LA Pressure** correlates with LV Pressure and thus, becomes the **closest approximation** of Preload

- **Can Measure** LA Pressure by using a Left Atrial Catheter

but tubes are tubes and series are series !!

- In Clinical Practice, **Pulmonary Capillary Wedge Pressure** is used as an index of LAP & LVEDP

PCWP = LAP = LVEDP *(best approximation)*

* But Remember, the relationship between LVEDP & LVEDVis **NOT Linear** !!

* PCWP is by definition an ESTIMATE of EDV& thus, an ESTIMATE of Preload

- At **Filling Pressures** of 15 - 18 mm Hg (PCWP), the ventricle operates on the very steep portion of the Diastolic Compliance Curve where further increases in PCWP lead to little change in EDV (and CO)

Issues: *Hyperdynamic Resuscitation*
Potential Injury / Relative Ischemia

- Also, the Relationship between PCWP & EDV is NOT Constant

- It is Affected by Changes in Compliance, Wall Thickness, HR, Ischemia, & Medications

- This is a **"One-Point-in-Time"** Effect

- Right-sided Filling Pressure: **CVP**
    – has been used as a rough estimate of LV Preload, but it may be an unreliable indicator of ventricular function *(especially in the critically ill patient)*

    – can be used to guide **Volume Status**
        • i.e. what is returning to the right atrium/right ventricle ?

    – may also be **useful** in patients with suspected cardiac tamponade or constrictive pericarditis

* Elevation of CVP to Equal PAD& PCWP

* **Square Root Sign** : characteristic RA waveform in patients with Constrictive Pericarditis

Afterload

the **impedance** *to LV Ejection and is usually estimated by* *the* **Systemic Vascular Resistance**

Remember: changes in afterload have **no effect** on the contractility of a normal heart

- The Normal Heart: SW performed at a given EDV is Insensitive to changes in SVR

- The Impaired Heart: Increasing afterload MAY decrease SW output for a given EDV, and thus impair myocardial performance

- when faced with this situation, if you reduce LV
  Impedance you may be able to increase CO !

    * Sodium Nitroprusside
    * Intra-Aortic Balloon Pump

$$SVR = \{(MABP - CVP)/CO\} \times 80$$

* MBAP (Mean Arterial Blood Pressure)

$$MBAP = DBP + [1/3\ (SBP - DBP)]$$

* SVR units: dynes-second/cm^5

Decreasing Afterload exchanges
Pressure Work for Flow Work

and serves to increase vital organ perfusion

Pressure Work...........................Flow Work

plus, since pressure work is more costly than flow work in terms of myocardial oxygen consumption, by decreasing afterload - you also decrease the overall energy requirement !

$$PVR = \{(MPAP - PWP)/CO\} \times 80$$

Remember:

1. Preload must be Optimized **PRIOR** to Afterload Reduction

2. A Low Arterial Pressure may preclude SVR Manipulation

3. **RV Afterload = PVR**
      * only a massive change in PVR can induce primary heart dysfunction

      * the vast majority of RV Failure is Secondary to LVF and usually responds to measures directed at the LV

      * Isolated RVF: Massive PE
                            Severe COPD
                            Isolated RV Infarct

Contractility

the inotropic state: an intrinsic property of myocardial muscle which is manifested as a greater force of contraction for a given preload

1. In terms of pressure & volume, the ventricle performs the same SW for a given EDV when the inotropic state is held constant.

2. When the inotropic state is augmented, more SW is produced at the same EDV

Clinically, this translates into **Increased CO & MAP** at a given Filling Pressure

* By increasing intropic state, you increase both Pressure Work & Flow Work - thus, the cost in myocardial oxygen consumption may be high

- An increased inotropic state may lead to a **delay** in recovery of function following myocardial injury!

- Inotropic Agents should only be used with caution & only AFTER other factors have been optimized!

   * Preload

   * Afterload

   * Heart Rate

Compliance & Elasticity

"compliance": the tendency of an object to return to it's original shape when it has been deformed or altered

(Compliance = change in Volume / change in Pressure)

1. The more elastic the muscle, the less it will be stretched by preload (i.e. the less compliant it is)

2. Elasticity is the **Reciprocal** of Compliance

Heart Rate

Heart Rate can *Influence* Cardiac Function in Several Ways:

Increasing the Contraction Frequency *limits* Diastolic Filling Time, Coronary Perfusion Time, & Reduces overall EDV

Increasing Rate *increases* Work Output from the ventricle per unit time at a given EDV [an Inotropic effect]

Increasing Rate *increases* Myocardial O2 Consumption

Bradycardia significantly *decreases* CO

Cardiac Physiology is based on a thorough understanding of the underlying mechanics !

C. Oxygen Calculations

The Oxygen Transport Variables:

Oxygen Content $[CaO_2]$
Oxygen Delivery $[DO_2]$
Oxygen Consumption $[VO_2]$
Extraction Ratio $[ER]$

Oxygen Content

the oxygen in the blood is either bound to hemoglobin or dissolved in plasma

- the sum of these two fractions is called the *Oxygen Content*

CaO_2 = the Content of Oxygen in Arterial Blood

> Hb = Hemoglobin (14 g/dl)
> SaO2 = Arterial Saturation (98%)
> PaO2 = Arterial PO2 (100 mmHg)

$CaO_2 = (1.3 \times Hb \times SaO_2) + (0.003 \times PaO_2)$
      amount carried by Hb   *amount dissolved in plasma*

$CaO_2 = (1.3 \times 14 \times 0.98) + (0.003 \times 100)$

$CaO_2 = 18.1$ ml/dl   (ml/dl = vol %; 18.1 vol %)

* at 100% Saturation, 1 g of Hb binds 1.3 ml of Oxygen !

* at 100% Saturation, 0.003 ml/mmHg of Oxygen is Dissolved in Plasma !

Note that the PaO_2 contributes *little* to the Oxygen Content !

- Despite it's popularity, the PaO_2 is NOT an important measure of arterial oxygenation !

- The SaO_2 is the more important blood gas variable for assessing the oxygenation of arterial blood !

the PaO_2 should be reserved for evaluating the efficiency of pulmonary gas exchange

Example # 1: *35 yr old male s/p GSW to Chest*

Pulse 126   BP 164 / 72
RR 26
Hb = 12
Hct = 36
ABG's: pH 7.38 / PaO_2 100 / $PaCO_2$ 32 / 96 % Sat

Question # 1: *What is this Patient's Oxygen Content ?*

Oxygen Delivery

DO_2: the Rate of Oxygen Tranport in the Arterial Blood

* it is the product of Cardiac Output & Arterial Oxygen Content

$$DO_2 = Q \times CaO_2$$

Cardiac Ouput (Q) can be "indexed" to body surface area

Normal C.I. : 2.5 - 3.5 L/min-m^2

By using a factor of 10, we can convert vol % to ml/s

$DO_2 = Q \times CaO_2$

$DO_2 = 3 \times (1.3 \times Hb \times SaO_2) \times 10$
$DO_2 = 3 \times (1.3 \times 14 \times .98) \times 10$
$DO_2 = 540$ ml/min-m^2

Normal Range: 520 - 720 ml/min-m^2

Example # 2: *35 yr old male s/p GSW to Chest*

Pulse 126   BP 164 / 72
RR 26
Hb = 12 / Hct = 36
ABG's: pH 7.38 / PaO_2 100 / $PaCO_2$ 32 / 96 %
Sat
C.I. = 2.86

Question # 2: *What is this Patient's Oxygen Delivery?*

Oxygen Consumption

oxygen uptake is the final step in the oxygen transport
pathway and it represents
the oxygen supply for tissue metabolism

The Fick Equation:

Oxygen Uptake is the Product of Cardiac Ouput and
the Arteriovenous Difference in Oxygen Content

$$VO_2 = Q \times [(CaO_2 - CvO_2)]$$

$VO_2 = Q \times (CaO_2 - CvO_2)$
$VO_2 = Q \times [(1.3 \times Hb) \times (SaO_2 - SvO_2) \times 10]$

$VO_2 = 3 \times [(1.3 \times 14) \times (.98 - .73) \times 10]$
$VO_2 = 3 \times [46]$
$VO_2 = 138 \ ml/min\text{-}m^2$

Normal VO2: 110 - 160 $ml/min\text{-}m^2$

Example # 3:   *35 yr old male s/p GSW to Chest*
Pulse 126   *BP 164 / 72*   *RR 26*
Hb = 12 / Hct = 36
ABG's: pH 7.38 / PaO_2 100 / $PaCO_2$ 32 / 96 % Sat
C.I. = 2.86
SvO_2 71 %

Question # 3: *What is this Patient's Oxygen Consumption
?*

Extraction Ratio

ER = *the fractional uptake of oxygen from the capillary bed*

O_2ER: derived as the Ratio of Oxygen Uptake to Oxygen Delivery

$$O_2ER = VO2 / DO2 \times 100$$

$$O_2ER = 130 / 540 \times 100$$

Normal Extraction

$O_2ER = 24\%$ (**22 - 32 %**)

Questions:
   1. **ER = 18 %**, what does this imply ?

   2. **ER = 40 %**, what does this imply ?

Example # 4: *35 yr old male s/p GSW to Chest*
Pulse 126   BP 164 / 72
RR 26
Hb = 12 / Hct = 36
ABG's: pH 7.38 / PaO_2 100 / $PaCO_2$ 32 / 96 %
Sat
C.I. = 2.86
SvO_2 71 %

Question # 4: *What is this Patient's Extraction Ratio?*

**the uptake of oxygen from the microcirculation is
a set point that is maintained by adjusting the
Extraction Ratio
to match changes in oxygen delivery**

*the ability to adjust O_2 Extraction can be impaired
in serious illness*

The Normal Response to a *Decrease in Blood Flow* is an
Increase in O_2 Extraction sufficient enough to *keep VO_2*
in the normal range

$VO_2 = Q \times Hb \times 13 \times (SaO2 - SvO2)$

$Q = 3$; $VO_2 = 3 \times 14 \times 13 \times (.97 - .73) = 110 \text{ ml/min-m}^2$

$Q = 1$; $VO_2 = 1 \times 14 \times 13 \times (.97 - .37) = 109 \text{ ml/min-m}^2$

- The Drop in Cardiac Index is BALANCED
  by an Increased $(SaO_2 - SvO_2)$ Difference and
  VO_2 remains Unchanged

- Note the drop in SvO_2 from 97 % to 37 % !!

- The Association between SvO_2 & O_2ER is the
  Basis for SvO_2 Monitoring

- The Ability to Adjust Extraction is a feature of all vascular beds except the Coronary Circulation & the Diaphragm !

The DO_2-VO_2 Curve

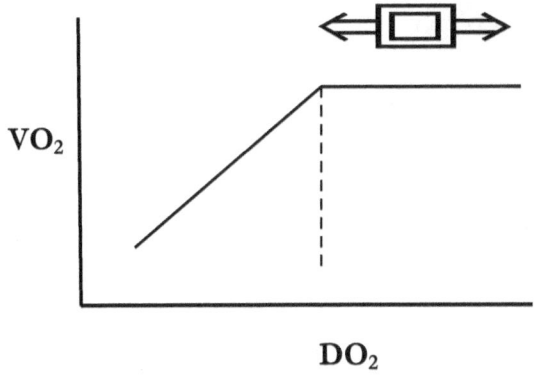

$$DO_2$$

- Flat Portion of the Curve
  - VO_2 Flow - Independent
  - O_2 Extraction varies in response to Blood Flow, keeping VO_2 Constant

- Linear Portion of the Curve
  - VO_2 Flow - Dependent
  - Indicates a defect in oxygen extraction from the microcirculation
  - Extraction is fixed and the VO_2 becomes directly dependent on Delivery

- Critical Level of Oxygen Delivery

- The Threshold DO_2 needed for Adequate Tissue Oxygenation
- If DO_2 falls below this level, oxygen supply will be sub-normal

Mixed Venous Oxygen

By rearranging the Fick Equation, the determinants of Venous Oxygen are:

$$VO2 = Q \times Hb \times 13 \times (SaO_2 - SvO_2)$$

$$SvO_2 = SaO_2 - (VO_2/Q \times Hb \times 13)$$

* the most prominent factor in determining SvO2 is **VO_2/Q**

Causes of a Low SvO_2:

> *Hypoxemia*
> *Increased Metabolic Rate*
> *Low Cardiac Output*
> *Anemia*

Another Point: Oximetry

Arterial Oxygen Saturation can be estimated but Venous Oxygen Saturation MUST be Measured !

* *Remember the shape of the Oxyhemoglobin Curve*

* The SaO$_2$ falls on the flat portion & can be safely estimated, while the Venous % Sat (68 - 77 % falls on the Steep Portion and can vary significantly even with small errors in estimation

In Critically-ill patients, augmenting the extraction ratio (in response to a change in oxygen delivery) **may not be possible.**

In these patients, the Venous Oxygen Levels may change **little** in response to changes in Cardiac Output.

Thus, the ***Relationship*** between CO(Q) and Mixed Venous Oxygen must be determined before using SvO$_2$ or PvO$_2$ to monitor changes in DO$_2$ or VO$_2$

The Transport Variables:

	Normal Range
Content [CaO$_2$]	16 - 19 vol %
Delivery [DO$_2$]	520 - 720 ml/min-m^2
Consumption [VO$_2$]	110 - 160 ml/min-m^2
Extraction Ratio [ER]	22 - 32 %
Mixed Venous PO$_2$	33 - 53 mmHg
Mixed Venous SO$_2$	68 - 77 %

** DO$_2$ & VO$_2$ are indexed to body surface area

D. The Chest: pneumothorax, hemothorax, effusions, and empyema

Pneumothorax

A collection of air within the pleural space

- transforms the potential space into a real one

- may lead to various degrees of respiratory compromise

- with progression, the intrapleural pressure may exceed atmospheric pressure creating a tension scenario

- impairs respiratory function

- decreases venous return to the right-side of the heart

General Management:

First   -   evacuate the air

Second -   address the underlying source

Third   -   promote pleural symphysis

Classification System

    A. Spontaneous Pneumothorax
- Primary
- Secondary

    B. Traumatic Pneumothorax
- Pulmonary source
- Tracheobronchial source
- Esophageal source

* Primary Spontaneous Ptx
- a disease of younger individuals *(15 - 35 yrs of age)*
- males > females
- tall, slim body habitus
- cigarette smoking implicated
- usual cause: <u>parenchymal blebs</u>
  - apex of the upper lobe
  - superior segment of the lower lobe

Question: when do you operate on a primary spontaneous pneumothorax ?

    C. Secondary Ptx *(due to underlying pulmonary disease)*
- COPD / Asthma / Cystic Fibrosis
- Immunocompromised Infections
  - Tb & Cocci
  - PCP *(becoming more common)*

    – Treatment: Closed Thoracostomy
- Water-seal
- Heimlich-Flutter Valve
- V.A.T.S.

Traumatic Ptx:

Parenchymal Injury vs. Tracheobronchial vs. Esophageal

    – Blunt or Penetrating
    – Iatrogenic
- central lines / thoracentesis / biopsy
- endotracheal tube placement *(esp. dual-lumen tubes !)*
- endoscopy / dilational techniques

    – Barotrauma
- Ventilation / blast injury / Boerhave's syndrome
    – Operative

- The Tension Ptx
  - *"path of least resistance"*
  - life-threatening emergency
  - Remember: **Large-bore needle, 2nd Intercostal Space followed by Thoracostomy**

- The Open Ptx: *sucking-chest wound*
  - intrinsic lung compliance creates complete collapse
  - 3-sided dressing

- thoracostomy **away** from the traumatic wound *(NEVER through the wound)*

- Treatment Options
  - Observation: Inpatient vs. Outpatient
  - Thoracostomy Drainage
    - 3rd Interspace/5th Interspace
    - Negative Suction/Water-seal
  - V.A.T.S.
  - Muscle-sparing Thoracotomy
  - Posterolateral & Anterolateral Thoracotomy

Complications of Tube Thoracostomy:

Hemorrhage
(laceration of intercostals artery, muscle or vein)

Parenchymal Laceration

Bronchopleural fistula

Cardiac injury

Subcutaneous tube placement (poor technique)

Intraperitoneal tube placement
(liver, stomach, colon, spleen injury)

Infection (cellulites, empyema)

Hemothorax

A collection of blood between the visceral and parietal pleura

- Causes of a Spontaneous Hemothorax
    - Pulmonary: bullous emphysema, PE, infarction, Tb, AVM's
    - Pleural: torn adhesions, endometriosis
    - Neoplastic: primary, metastatic *(melanoma)*
    - Blood Dyscrasias: thrombocytopenia, hemophilia, anticoagulation
    - Thoracic Pathology: ruptured aorta, dissection
    - Abdominal Pathology: pancreatic pseudocyst, hemoperitoneum

The Pathophysiologic Process
- the accumulation of pleural blood forms a stable clot
- overall ventilation & oxygenation becomes impaired
    - mechanical compression of the lung parenchyma
    - mediastinal shift
    - flattening of the hemidiaphragm
- over time, the clot is partially-absorbed, leaving behind loculated fluid and fibrinous septations
- macro-fibrin deposition begins to provide a structural framework

- this "peel" slowly contracts to entrap the underlying lung

Goal of Treatment: *to remove the pleural blood and allow for complete lung re-expansion*

- General Management Options
  - thoracentesis: *bedside / ultrasound-guided / C.T.-guided*
  - thoracostomy drainage: *the mainstay*
  - thorascopic surgery: *less than 2 wks. & use a 30-degree scope*
  - thoracotomy: *massive hemothorax / instability / chronic hemothorax*
  - local fibrinolytic therapy: *urokinase (1000 IU/ml) in 150 solution*

- Often, there is an accompanying pneumothorax
  - Dual Chest Tube Management
    - Superior-Apical: Ptx
    - Diaphragmatic-posterior: Htx
    - Consider targeted-drainage into a loculated collection
  - All tubes to negative suction with protective water-seal
  - Prophylactic antibiotics are indicated while the tubes are in
  - Chest tubes removed: 100 -150 cc's/day

An undrained hemothorax increases the risk of empyema & fibrothorax!

- Large collections should be drained slowly to minimize the development of *re-expansion-pulmonary-edema ["R.E.E.P."]*

]

- Computed tomography is the diagnostic procedure of choice

Pleural Effusions

An accumulation of fluid in the pleural space

Pathophysiology:

    altered pleural membrane permeability
    decreased intravascular oncotic pressure
    increased pleural capillary hydrostatic pressure
    lymphatic obstruction
    abnormal sites of entry

Clinical Features:
    Pain and breathlessness
    Dullness to percussion
    Diminished or absent breath sounds
    Decreased or absent vocal resonance
    Decreased or absent tactile vocal fremitus
    Egophony at level of meniscus

Diagnostic Approach:
    Confirm by Radiographic Imaging
    Posteroanterior chest radiograph
    Lateral decubitus chest radiographs
    Ultrasound *(loculations)*
    CT Scan

Once presence is confirmed radiographically, then perform Thoracentesis to differentiate: Transudate vs. Exudate

Laboratory Studies:

Cell count and differential
Gram stain, culture and sensitivity
Cytology
Protein, LDH
Other-glucose, amylase, afb

Criteria for Exudate:
fluid-to-serum ratio of total protein > 0.5
fluid-to-serum ratio of LDH > 0.6
fluid LDH concentration > 2/3 upper limit
of normal for serum LDH

Transudative Effusions result from:
Increased capillary hydrostatic pressure
Reduced colloid osmotic pressure

Transudative Effusions, Differential Diagnosis:

Heart failure
(usually presents as a bilateral effusion)
Hepatic cirrhosis *(usually is Right-sided)*
Nephrotic Syndrome *(due to hypoalbuminemia)*
Ascites *(usually is Right-sided)*
Constrictive pericardial disease
SVC obstruction
Pulmonary Embolism

Exudative Effusions result from:
Disruption of pleural membrane
Obstruction of lymphatic drainage

Exudative Effusions, Differential Diagnosis:
Infections *(parapneumonic, t.b.)*
Malignant disorders
(primary or metatstatic disease)
Vasculitic disease *(R.A., S.L.E.)*
Gastrointestinal disease
(pancreatitis, esophageal rupture, hepatic abscess)
Pulmonary Embolism

Treatment depends on the underlying
pathophysiologic process...

If exudative, usually thoracostomy tube drainage.

THE GOAL is to prevent an empyema
or a "trapped lung"

Empyema Thoracis

An Accumulation of Pus in the Pleural Cavity

- 1-2 % incidence in the pediatric population
- Up to 18 % in immunocompromised adults
- General Management
    - Appropriate Antibiotic Coverage
    - Thoracostomy Drainage

  – Streptokinase / Urokinase
  – Surgical Intervention - Decortication

The Stages of Empyema:

Stage I - *"Exudative"*
  • sterile pleural fluid develops secondary to inflammation without fusion of the pleura

Stage II - *"Fibrinopurulent"*
  • a fibrinous peel develops on both pleural surfaces limiting lung expansion

Stage III - *"Organizing"*
  • in-growth of capillaries & fibroblasts into the fibrinous peel

Treatment: *AVOID !!!*

aggressive drainage....
early VATS

<u>NOTES</u>